A P Better and Slimmer You: Body Building for Women

Discover Little Known Secrets on Body Building for Women

By: Yvette Green

Bodybuilding For Women

Publisher Notes

Disclaimer

Bodybuilding For Women

Always read all information provided by the manufacturers' product labels before using their products. The author and publisher are not responsible for claims made by manufacturers.

Table of Contents

DEDICATION

This is dedicated to my daughter who has helped me a lot with this book.

Introduction

We all understand that boosting and maintaining ample muscle mass is one of the very best methods to keep body fat at bay and to improve overall fitness, particularly as we age. We also know weightlifting is the very best way to develop muscular tissue mass.

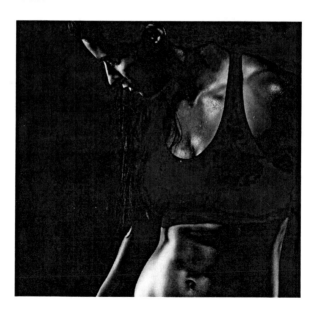

Women, Cardio and Over Weightlifting

Even with a lot of research supporting the benefits of body building and strength training, most women still select cardio over weightlifting. Perhaps they're concerned with thoughts of "expanding" or bulking up. Ladies have seen way too many beefy guys grunting it out in the gym and fear that if they pick up a dumbbell they'll start to appear like them.

This can occur, although it's remarkably unusual and rare. For most women, "this isn't really possible," says personal trainer and fitness professional Yvette Green, "Ladies have way too much estrogen in their hormone make-up." Time and again studies have revealed women who keep a routine of mild strength training, benefit with a long list of health benefits and advantages.

Enhancing your strength will certainly make you far less dependent on others for assistance in everyday living. Tasks will be less complicated; carrying your children,

10

groceries and laundry will certainly not push you to the maximum. With increased muscle strength, daily duties and regular workouts will be much less likely to induce injury. Research studies conclude mild weightlifting could increase a woman's strength by thirty to fifty percent.

Research also shows that women can develop their strength at the very same rate as guys. Analysts found that unlike guys, females generally do not bulk up from bodybuilding or weight training, considering that compared to guys, women have ten to thirty times less of the hormones which induce muscular tissue hypertrophy. You will, however, improve beneficial muscle tone.

The Bodybuilding Advantage

Improves your athletic potential

Bodybuilding improves your athletic potential. Golfers could significantly raise their driving power. Bikers are able to ride for longer periods with less fatigue. Skiers enhance technique and minimize injury.

Whatever sport you play, strength training and weight lifting has been shown to improve total efficiency and stamina.

The average woman who weight trains a couple of times a week for two months can gain two pounds of muscular tissue and shed three and a half pounds of fat deposits. As your lean muscular tissue increases, so does your metabolism and you burn even more calories all day. Generally speaking, for every pound of muscle you gain, you burn thirty-five to fifty additional calories on a daily basis. That being said, weight lifting can actually burn up unwanted fats.

Improve spinal bone mineral density
Research has found that weightlifting can improve spinal bone mineral density, and boost bone structure by thirteen percent in six months. This, paired with sufficient dietary calcium, will help protect women against the weakening of bones or osteoporosis. Bodybuilding doesn't just create stronger muscular tissues, but also constructs more powerful connective tissues and boosts joint stability.

This works as support for the joints and aids to prevent injury. The latest research revealed that strengthening the lower back had an eighty percent success rate in eliminating or relieving back discomforts. Various other investigations additionally suggested that weightlifting could relieve the pain of osteoarthritis and support joints.

Enhance your heart strength

Body Building can enhance your heart strength in numerous ways. Training can decrease LDL ("bad cholesterol"), thus boosting the HDL ("good cholesterol"), and decrease blood pressure. When cardiovascular exercise is added, these advantages are maximized.

Additionally, weight training can help the body process sugar, which can highly minimize the threat of diabetes, an increasing problem for women and men as they age. Weightlifting can help boost glucose utilization in the body by twenty-three percent in four months.

Females in their 70s and 80s can also develop strength from weightlifting or body building, especially with professional help and assistance. Research reveals that strength improvements are feasible at any age. Nevertheless, the training should be managed by an expert.

Enhance psychological or mental wellness
You will likewise improve psychological or mental wellness, which helps to fight anxiety and depression. Studies discovered that ten weeks of weight training can reduce nervous breakdown symptoms much more effectively than counseling can. Women who train frequently have stated that they feel more capable as a result of their program.

CHAPTER 1
-
The Physiology of the Female Muscle

Physiological Differences between Male and Female

In addition to the obvious distinctions between the sexes, some considerable and ingrained physical variables additionally divide the females from the males.

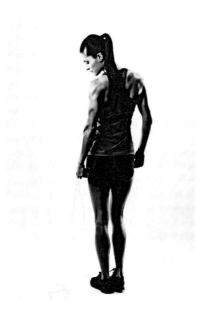

Understand that the female body likes making use of fat deposits for energy needed by the body, while the male body commonly burns superior amounts of carbohydrates, in addition to some fat deposits and healthy protein.

When women exercise for strength and size, their physical body activates the same number of Type I (also known as slow-twitch, or aerobic) muscle fibers and Type II (aka fast-twitch, or power) fibers, whereas the male who lifts weights establishes Type II fibers disproportionately.

Men, who take part in an identical exercise as women, will demonstrate more indicators of catabolism and muscle breakdown right after finishing the routine.

Typically, the muscle tissue of males and females coincide and respond in a comparable way. However, males create more muscle mass than females. The abilities of both sexes vary, which is why the development of muscle groups depend on your exercise program and way of life.

Muscle Development Differences

Based on 2004 research released by the American Physiology Society, the skeletal muscles of men build faster as opposed to the female skeletal muscular tissues. Women have the advantage of faster recovery and have more ability to resist fatigue.

Estrogen-B appears to play a factor in muscle contractile rate, which makes males much more efficient in creating power and females more efficient in healing. The male releases testosterone which is extremely essential in building muscle. It explains why men develop larger muscles than females.

Differences in Muscle Structure

Men and women's muscle tissues are nearly identical, yet vary depending upon genetics and their routine activities.

There are three major types of muscle fibers:

- Type I fibers
- Type IIa fibers

  - Type IIb fibers

According to a post released in *FASEB Journal*, these fibers are also called slow twitch fibers and fast twitch fibers. Slow twitch fibers are necessary for endurance and conditioning while fast twitch fibers are essential for energy. Males often have quicker twitch muscle fibers. This is the main reason why males are more powerful and females are much more resistant to fatigue.

Differences in Muscle Strength
Based on a 1999 research study released in *Journal of Applied Physiology*, males have more skeletal muscle mass than women. This is the reason most males are stronger. More muscle mass equals more power.

Nevertheless, as you get heavier, skeletal muscle composition begins to decrease, so it is vital to maintain a healthy weight to ensure muscle mass stays proportionate. Females can also develop their skeletal muscles to improve durability. However, females still have to remain within the suitable weight range to keep durability proportionate to body size.

Differences in Response to Training

Research shown in *Experimental Physiology* demonstrates that males and females react similarly to training and exercise. Nevertheless, females are a lot more resistant to fatigue because they have more slow-moving twitch fibers and bodily hormones like estrogen. Males have more energy and power yet are much less immune as a result of the higher volume of fast twitch fibers in their bodies.

Females often participate in cardiovascular training which is why they have improved slow twitch fibers. Males tend to lift weights and do brief, yet highly effective, cardio physical exercises, therefore developing their fast twitch fibers more.

The fact is that training for females does not vary all that much from durability training for men. Though men normally produce testosterone, giving them an advantage in acquiring a "ripped" look, there are numerous workouts that both sexes can do to increase their muscles.

Without using anabolic steroids or some kind of testosterone supplements, females will never have the ability to obtain the bulky results that men do with bodybuilding exercises. They can perform the exact same physical exercises, raising the exact same weights to tone muscles and add muscle mass to their body.

Strength Training Exercises For Women

Many women, who want to strength train for toned muscles, know that being stuck in the cardio room using the treadmill is not sufficient. Rather, women must perform proven exercises to achieve better and toned muscles.

Curls

No matter what your gender is, curls are a wonderful way to work out the arms. Sadly, women do not have the ability to build more muscle mass. However, it is in curling weights that women can tone the muscle in their arms

Tricep pulldowns

You are going to be concentrating on toning your arms through the use of tricep pulldowns. You will not add more muscle mass to your arms, but women can keep their triceps from becoming saggy by doing this exercise.

Squats

While men will enhance the muscle mass of their upper legs with squats, ladies will simply tone theirs with squat exercises. This move is also beneficial for toning calves, hamstrings and glutes.

Bench press

The fundamental weightlifting workout is the bench press. In addition to adding muscle mass to the pectoral muscular tissues, it also targets the biceps and triceps. Women will not wind up with bulky pectoral muscular tissues if they decide to do this physical exercise, it will lead to toned pectoral muscles.

Amplifying Women's Strength Training

Women will have to do more strategic workouts if they want to get more results from their routine. A good note to remember is that men make use of their all-natural testosterone to bulk up, while ladies focus on toning muscle mass.

However, for women searching for that added muscle mass, it is essential to make changes to a regular diet plan. A very good example is to add eggs to daily meals. Eggs are known to enhance hypertrophy in both sexes.

Hypertrophy is the increase in tissue surrounding muscles. Likewise, it is necessary that adequate lean meats are consumed. This assists in burning fat deposits and will add muscle mass to the body during exercises.

Strength training for men and women is not all that different when it comes right down to it. The real difference lies in the results.

No matter their gender, it is essential to understand what the body is capable of before beginning strength training. Establish realistic goals and start accomplishing them.

CHAPTER 2
-
Toning, Shaping and Sculpting

Everyone has a picture in their minds of how their body will look when they're in shape. Some want to fit back into their favorite clothes, or show off their washboard abs, others want to wear a bikini to the beach with complete self-confidence.

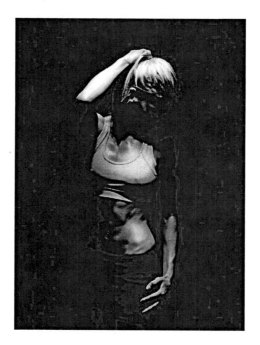

Others are satisfied when looking at defined abs and pecs in the mirror, or seeing strong, toned shoulders or legs in our reflections. While everyone's goals are different, practically everyone wants to look toned, sculpted and shaped.

Toning Indications

What does "toned", "muscle toning", or "shaping" actually mean? Is it different from "bulking" up? When most people say they want to "tone up" what they usually mean is that they wish to become leaner. Essentially, they would like to lose fat and have muscle definition, but not muscle mass.

In the health and fitness niche, there is no universal definition for toning. Instead, toning is a term used to describe the goal and target, which generally results from a combination of weight-lifting and fat-burning.

Toning and Sculpting Towards Musculature

Toning and sculpting exercises are physical routines generally used to develop and improve the overall look of the body. These are workouts with the objective of improving the figure with a huge emphasis on definition. Toning indicates leanness in the body, with reduced levels of physical body fats, without an emphasis on increased muscle size.

Women want to tone their legs, abs, arms, back, perhaps their entire body. Whichever body part you want to work on, you must know about toning. You should know the best muscle toning exercises and all of the tips and methods. Appearing "toned, shaped or sculpted" is a common health and fitness objective, particularly for women.

Bulking up is generally a man's preference. Although there is no strict definition, bulking up implies adding a great deal of muscle mass to the physical body and possibly reducing one's physical body fat. Toning, on the other hand, typically describes to have lesser quantities of body fat and some visible muscular tissue, but not massive muscular tissues.

Exactly how can you be toned, shaped or sculpted?

You may wonder if "toning, shaping or sculpting" is possible. Is muscle tone merely a misconception? Is there really a way to tone your body? Will you ever see the results you want? Tone is certainly real and definitely possible.

Toning is having some muscle with a much lower body fat percentage on your body, which gives definition. The more muscles you have and less fatty tissue covering it, becomes "toned" and "defined".

Whenever a person says they want to tone up, they're saying they would like to see more of their muscle compared to what they currently have. To accomplish it requires one of the following, lose the fat or build more muscle, but the very best bet will be a combination of both.

Important Factors Regarding Muscle Toning, Shaping, Sculpting and Bulking Up

Lifting lighter weights will tone your body and lifting heavy weights will bulk you up.

For many years, males and females have always believed that when you use heavy weights it bulks you up, which is not totally true. This misconception is what makes a lot of people fear heavy weights. On the other hand, there is some truth that lighter weights and more repetitions increases stamina. Thus, lighter weights will not assist you "tone" better compared to massive weights.

Since bigger weights increase the toughness of your muscles and improve your metabolic process and burn fat deposits, lifting heavier weights with less repetitions—8 to 12 reps and working till you're fatigued—is more apt to help you reach your toning goals than lifting lighter weights. Additionally, this workout is quicker compared to lifting lighter weights for longer amounts of time.

Building muscle and bulking up are one and the same

You have been steering clear of weights because you assumed that building muscle means you'll increase mass. When you put up weights that are challenging, you are producing micro-tears in the muscular tissue fibers. These splits are then mended by the physical body; this is where soreness and discomfort comes from! Because of this, muscles end up being more powerful and a little bit bigger.

Thus, adding a little muscle and lowering your fatty tissue really makes you look leaner, not larger, since muscle is much denser than fat. If you intend to mass up, you have to keep that thought in mind.

Weightlifters spend hours and hours in the gym, lifting very heavy weights, along with a meticulous diet rich in protein, which is why they can really increase in size.

The average person's exercise and diet regimen and a calorie-controlled diet don't produce the same results

Lifting light weights won't help you get stronger

The secret to obtaining a strong and toned body isn't really about how much weight you're lifting. It is about working your muscles to fatigue, where you absolutely can't raise the weight for another repetition. One study showed that when subjects lifted light weights they engaged as much muscular tissue as those lifting heavy weights.

Nonetheless, the time it takes to reach exhaustion with light weights is much longer compared to the moment it takes to reach exhaustion with heavier weights. So, if you're like many people and time is crucial, it makes more sense to go heavy.

Women and men should lift weights differently

This happens all the time at the gym; it's quite typical to see females raise 3 to 5 pound dumbbells to do biceps curls while men get the 20 pound set to do the same exercise. Although men are genetically more powerful compared to ladies, they aren't that much more powerful.

A lot of females have the tendency to adhere to the weight devices or basic leg-work that target the back side and abs, I'm talking about those vanity muscles, while the men are more likely to be exercising with barbells or using weights and most often concentrating on their vanity muscular tissues as well, such as the arms and chest.

Everybody has different targets, but if you truly intend to slim down and get lean–it does not matter if you call it toning or bulking–men and women alike need a strength-training strategy in place that engages every major muscle in the body.

It is imperative to use heavy enough weights so the last two repetitions are very difficult to complete. This is when the body is truly challenged enough to alter, expand and adjust, making both men and women stronger and leaner. Lifting in this way also helps you to lose unwanted body fat.

Certain forms of exercise build long, lean muscles

A lot of exercises lengthen and create lean muscles. But the fact is no kind of workout makes them "longer" because your muscles do not and will not react to exercise that way, it's just not how muscle cells work. Muscular tissues have a maximum length because they are attached to your bones.

A wide range of movements and workouts can help you strengthen your muscles without making them larger. You can develop a bunch of muscle toughness and strength without increasing in size or girth.

In addition, exercises such as Yoga, Pilates, dancing and barre classes can help increase flexibility, boost joint movement, and enhance your posture, making you feel and look taller.

CHAPTER 3
-
The Body Builder's Diet

In muscle building, a proper diet plan is equally as important as exercise. The bodybuilding diet is similar for men and women. You need to consider a lot of factors when creating a meal plan. A terrific muscle building diet is a key element that will determine how successful you are in your workout program.

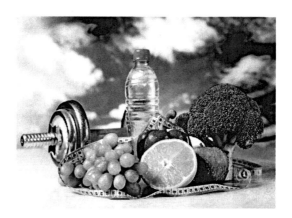

Training without healthy and nutritious food is like rowing against the waves. At best, you will remain the same, or progress a little bit, but ultimately, you'll get nowhere.

A Definition of Diet

Generally, people associate the word "diet" with days of hunger and discomfort. They think not eating a meal or two in a day, is all they need to do to lose those unwanted pounds. But that is not the correct definition. The word diet simply describes our daily meal choices.

Even if you don't think you are on a diet, you are actually following one as we speak. Whether you consume candy, eat oatmeal, or drink water all day–that is your diet. Most importantly, you don't have to starve to have a good and healthy diet.

The Difference between Male and Female Bodybuilders

A lot of bodybuilding diets were developed with men in mind and that is why their diet plans are slightly different than women's. Females do not metabolize fatty tissue as quickly as men, do not create the same testosterone levels, and also have a more difficult time acquiring muscles, so their diet is different.

Because of distinct differences in metabolic rates, women have unique dietary needs. A normal diet consists of three meals: breakfast, lunch and dinner. A bodybuilding diet consists of six smaller sized meals eaten every three hours. Keep in mind that a meal is not a snack. Every meal should have a certain percentage of protein, carbs and good fats.

Try increasing the amount of carbohydrates early in the day, and decrease them with each subsequent meal. Carbohydrates are your energy meals; eat a dish that is rich in carbs right before you work out. Protein is equal throughout the day because your body needs consistent amounts. Make sure your proteins are lean.

Lastly, your body burns fat while you're asleep, suggesting the majority of your fat consumption must be later in the day. You should cycle the amount of calories you consume each day. It will keep your body from becoming used to any kind of certain calorie count.

The number of calories consumed will need to be modified to match your metabolic rate. It is necessary to consume calories as you burn, or else your body stores those excess calories as fat deposits. Since women have the tendency to store more fat than men, it is essential in a body building diet to eat much less fat and cholesterol. When shopping, look for the low-fat and low-cholesterol versions of food.

General Guidelines for the Ideal Diet Plan

Before we discuss the recommended diet for women who want to lose fat and gain lean muscle, let's look at some general diet standards. This guideline will assist you as you create your own healthy and balanced diet. Take into consideration all the factors and I'm sure you'll formulate a great plan, to get the fantastic body you've always wanted.

Calorie Control

The biggest factor is calories in versus calories out; your overall calories will determine if you lose or gain weight. Consuming a lot of calories results in fat gain. But if you don't eat enough calories, you won't obtain lean muscle. Establishing a set calorie target and counting the amount of calories you consume every day is essential to losing fatty tissue and gaining lean muscle.

Macronutrient Control

While overall calorie intake is important in a diet, the ratio of healthy protein to carbohydrates to fats can determine whether the weightloss is muscle or fat. A diet with 80% of calories from carbohydrates, 10% from healthy protein, and 10% from fat will certainly have different results compared to a diet regimen containing 40% of calories from carbs, 40% from protein, and 20% from fatty tissue.

Stay Hydrated

You need to consume lots of water. You should drink at least eight glasses or sixty-four ounces of water daily. Consuming enough water provides hydration along with helping you feel full without adding calories. Sometimes people mistake thirst for hunger. Because of this, staying hydrated could help to eliminate overeating. You should keep a bottle of water with you at all times.

Quality Assurance Or Control

Choose fresh, balanced meals over pre-packaged, processed foods. Packaged foods are loaded with preservatives, especially sodium and saturated fats, and frequently have high quantities of sugars. You will be amazed at how fast you can lose fat just by packing your meals from home instead of purchasing fast food or packaged meals. You can also save a lot of money by doing this!

Insulin Control

Insulin is the "storage space" hormone. When it is produced it reduces fat burning. By choosing reduced GI carbohydrates you manage the hormone secretion and increase weight loss. Steady blood glucose levels can also improve energy and one's state of mind.

Diets lower in glucose; can cause leaner muscle gains with little or no fat gain.

Adequate Healthy Proteins

In order to obtain lean muscle you need to eat sufficient healthy protein to maintain the development of brand-new muscle. You may not be used to eating the amount of healthy protein our suggested diet regimen suggests, but once you get in the groove you won't have any trouble and will certainly enjoy how satisfying it feels.

Necessary Fats

Important greasy acids (EFAs) are vital for your body to properly function. Dietary fats got a bad rap because of the diet fads of the 80s and 90s, which advertised eating as little fat as possible, but in reality EFAs are required by the body and are part of a healthy diet. Consuming fats does not equal getting fat.

As a matter of fact, many EFAs help support the fat burning process and keep a body lean. Do not be afraid to eat good fats. EFAs are not the opponent. Also, make sure to supplement yourself with a high quality EFA product, such as Scivation Fundamental FA.

A Basic Diet Plan Template

This is a great diet plan and recommended meal regimen. As long as you adhere to this and commit to exercise I'm certain you'll get the body you want. You must split your protein between each of your meals. About 2/3 to 3/4 of your carbs need to be consumed around 4-6 hours after your exercise.

For breakfast: About 15% Of Complete Caloric Intake:

- 1/3 of starchy carbohydrates (oatmeal, whole wheat or grain bread, etc.)
- 2/3 of healthy protein (eggs, milk, lean meat)
- Small portion of good fats (fish oil, olive oil, nuts, etc.)
- Your selection of fruits or vegetables
- Water or Green Tea

For Lunch or Mid-Day Meal (like for the time after or before exercise):

- 1/2 of starchy carbs (Whole grains, noodles, whole grain bread, cereals, cooked potatoes, etc.)
- 1/2 of lean protein (Egg whites, tuna, other fish, lean red meat, skim milk, etc.)
- Marginal fats
- Any sort of Fruits & Veggies from the listing
- Water or Green Tea

Dinner or Supper or Also Called Pre-Bed Meal:

- 1/2 of starchy carbs (Whole grains, pasta, whole grain bread, oats, baked potatoes, etc.)
- 1/2 of lean protein (Egg whites, tuna, other fish, lean red meat, skim milk, etc.)
- Small serving of good fat
- Any Fruits & Vegetables from the list
- Water or Green Tea

Health Supplements

There are a few supplements which are recommended to help in your diet and body building and, if possible, they should all be used. These are the essential supplements to be considered and added to your diet for optimal body building results.

Fish Oil for your healthy metabolism. The oil also provides a host of other health benefits. You should take at least three grams of fish oil daily and multi-vitamins for the essential minerals and vitamins needed by the body. Creatinine is the element that helps your body in muscle loss prevention when cutting occurs. It also boosts performance and recovery.

Take note that it will cause some water retention in the muscles. Whey Protein is a must for every post workout shake; it is beneficial when taken occasionally throughout the day, as it can help boost protein synthesis due to its fast absorption.

With all these guidelines and tips for your diet plan, you'll eat healthier with or without heavy exercises.

Bodybuilding For Women

CHAPTER 4
-
Increasing Protein Synthesis

"To grow or maintain muscle, you should consume 1 gram of protein per pound of bodyweight." This statement makes me shake my head. I cannot believe people buy into this. Trust me; I've done my research on this, not to mention my qualifications entitle me to offer my professional opinion on the matter.

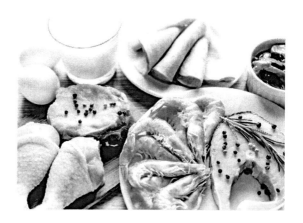

The Benefits and Requirements of Protein for Active Women

This is just ridiculous! I said out loud while I was reading a famous diet book for women. The book states cereal, yogurt, a glass of juice and coffee for breakfast! I was looking for protein! Where did the protein-rich diet go? I agree that yogurt has protein; however it's not sufficient enough to keep the nutrition, satiation and energy that the active woman requires.

I think it's time to set the record straight. We need to take these old misleading myths and put them in the trash. Women NEED protein, period. And every woman needs to know this.

The Protein Issue

Sadly, when it comes to a woman's diet, protein is not given enough importance. A lot of people seem to believe women don't need much protein in their diets, but I am here to tell you that we do.

Protein is made up of amino acids, the foundation of many cells in the body, including muscular tissue. Specific amino acids are "essential", meaning the body can not make them and they need to be obtained from food.

When working out, our body breaks down muscle tissue. In order to fix the muscle cells, gain lean mass and end up being more powerful, you must replenish proteins to provide the amino acids required for healing.

Where will it obtain the needed amino acids lacking in your daily diet if you are not going to provide it?

All of that hard work will go to waste! In addition to needing them to recuperate from heavy workouts, amino acids and protein are essential for a lot of reasons, like:

- It helps in the proper function of the immune system
- It promotes healthy connective tissue which includes hair and nails
- It helps boost energy levels

Now that we know why healthy protein is essential, let's see how much healthy protein a woman needs.

The daily allowance of healthy protein for sedentary adults is 0.8 grams per kg of bodyweight (0.8 g/kg) or 0.36 grams per pound of bodyweight (0.36 g/lb). The recommended protein proportion is the same for both men and women. But how about energetic females, do they need more healthy protein compared to inactive females? The response is a definite YES.

Facts about Protein

The International Society of Sports Nutrition recently reported their position on protein intake:

1. Extensive study gives support to the idea that individuals engaged in routine training need more nutritional protein than less active people.
2. 1.4 to 2.0 g/kg intakes of protein each day for physically energetic

individuals may boost the training adaptations to exercise training.

3. When protein intake is a part of a balanced diet, these levels are not harmful to kidneys in healthy, active individuals.

4. While it is possible for physically active individuals to get their daily protein requirements through regular diet, extra protein in various forms are a smart way to ensure athletes get enough.

5. Different types and qualities of protein can influence amino acid bioavailability following healthy protein supplements. The supremacy of one healthy protein kind over another in regards to maximizing recuperation and/or training adaptations continues to be convincingly shown.

6. Suitably timed healthy protein consumption is an essential part of a total exercise training program, vital for proper healing, immune

function, and the growth and upkeep of lean physical body mass.

7. Under specific conditions, particular amino acid supplements, such as branched-chain amino acids (BCAA's), might boost physical exercise performance and recuperation from exercise." (Campbell et al, 2007).

We can assume that active women could benefit from consuming 2 grams/kg of bodyweight, which equals 1 gram/lb of bodyweight. For a 150 pound woman, this indicates that she needs 150 grams of healthy protein per day. Preferably your protein needs to be spaced out throughout the day. This would be 30 grams of protein per meal if you ate five meals a day.

Let's look at an example. The proteins will be listed but not the fats and carbs since they differ depending on a person's diet regimen and targeted goals.

- Meal 1: 1 Cup Egg Whites

- Meal 2: 1.5 Scoops PGN Whey Sensible (Whey Protein)
- Meal 3: 4 oz. Chicken
- Post-Workout:
- Meal 4: 1.5 Scoops PGN Whey Sensible/Whey Protein
- Meal 5: 4 oz. Fish (Tilapia or Salmon)

***Take note that each of the protein amounts listed above is about 30 grams protein.

Ideal Sources of Protein:

- Eggs, especially egg whites
- Lean beef
- Chicken
- Turkey
- Fishes like tuna, salmon, tilapia, halibut and mahi mahi
- Protein Powders like whey
- Tofu

There is no reason you can't reach your protein goals daily! With top quality, reduced carbohydrate, healthy protein powders, it is easy to make a quick shake and please your sweet tooth at the same time.

Women who want to progress in the gym and reach their goal of the perfect lean body need to know that eating protein is essential and they must not listen to anyone who says they do not need it!

CHAPTER 5
-
Beginning A Simple Resistance Training Program

Resistance Training Program

Resistance exercise is also called strength training, and it is done to improve muscle strength, bone strength development and metabolism improvement.

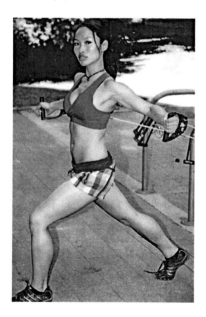

It is essential that you build strong muscles, considering they can help you to perform daily activities with ease and fewer restraints.

Resistance exercise induces the development of small healthy proteins in the muscle cells, which will consequently improve your muscular tissues' capacity to produce force.

Normally, a resistance workout is made up many kinds of exercises primarily done on equipment made for developing particular muscle groups. A regular exercise routine lasts for about half an hour, and you could do one or many sets of each exercise. In one set of a workout, you could do 8 to 15 repetitions.

If you want to see development in muscle and mass within a shorter time, it is advised that you schedule two or three workouts weekly. You will see the biggest improvement in the first couple of months of training.

The Importance of Resistance in Body Building

Resistance exercise benefits your body in many ways.

1. It causes a rise in the levels of high-density lipoprotein, or excellent cholesterol levels, and this will certainly contribute to much better cardiovascular health.

2. It influences your physical composition in a positive way. Given that muscle burn calories, an increase in muscle mass will certainly minimize fat and boost your metabolic rate. Therefore, resistance exercise is an effective way to lose and maintain weight.

3. It is understood that this type of workout can raise the amount of bone minerals in your body, and can make you less susceptible to osteoporosis. If you are over the age of 35, your body will experience progressive loss of muscular tissue mass, and without

exercise you will end up being weaker as you get older.

4. If you perform resistance training regularly, you could decelerate the loss of muscle mass. In a recent study, men and women in their 70s and 80s received resistance training for ten weeks and researchers observed that their muscle durability, agility and mobility had noticibly improved after the training. Numerous doctors order their elderly patients to do resistance physical exercise at least twice a week.

5. Recent studies have also revealed that resistance training might be more proper than aerobic exercises in enhancing physical image and self-esteem. One factor for this is that resistance training supplies more immediate outcomes. After training for a brief time period, you will observe that your muscular tissues have grown and become more toned.

Everyone should check with their doctors before performing this type of exercise, especially if they have medical problems or orthopedic concerns.

Obviously, some workouts are not recommended to individuals if they have certain health issues or they experience joint discomfort with specific physical exercises.

Although a variety of activity is suggested for healthy and well balanced individuals, workouts using a maximum range of motion without discomfort or pain are suggested from professionals.

For example, the depth of a squat will depend on the health of the knees. If one is unable to support their body weight, they could initially execute a fifty percent squat until they are strong enough to perform it fully.

Strength or resistance training is a vital workout for almost everyone. Besides the evident muscle-building, it can help you to burn even more calories and make bones stronger.

The Right Way to Start Resistance Training

There is a lot of confusion of where to begin in a resistance training program. If you need a jumpstart to a routine, then the right thing to do is to educate yourself, and have the will to begin. Novice or not, the resistance training will help you to build your whole new self.

Certified trainers often come across people who have no clue as to how to start lifting weights. When it comes to lifting weights, it is not all about pulling or pressing huge quantities of iron in a gym.

It does not mean that you've got to be so sore the following day that walking hurts. We need to change our minds about what "lifting weights" really means. Both men and women have had misconceptions and some are a little afraid of lifting weights.

A safe weight training program is something that will help you reach your fitness goals. Resistance training is a key ingredient when you want to lose fat, as well as keep muscles in top shape.

The very first step for an optimal resistance workout plan is to start slow; each exercise will help to increase stamina. The following regimen can be performed either in the comfort of your home or outside, in your backyard or at the park.

Even if you don't have a yard or room in your house, a lot of neighborhoods have playgrounds where these exercises could be performed. Keep in mind that resistance training is for your benefit, for your physical and mental health.

Resistance Exercise Methods

There are primarily three different means to do resistance exercises:

- weight machines
- free weights
- calisthenics

Weight Machines

When you are using weight equiptment, you choose the weight you would like to lift by including or removing plates for your workout regimen, but your motions are dictated by the machine you use.

Free weights

Free weights allow you to perform many exercises to work out the entire body when you are lifting.

Calisthenics

Calisthenics are carried out without the use of weights, and they include physical exercises such as pushups, situps and chinups.

In these workouts, your body weight is the resistance. All that being said, resistance training is a workout that anyone can do daily.

CHAPTER 6
-
Sample Routine and Daily Workout Schedule

The Weekly Workout Program

As we said in the previous chapters, women need to lift heavy, challenging weights in order to get targeted lean muscles. Lifting weights will not trigger women to get bulky and huge like men, since women do not generate a portion of the testosterone that men do.

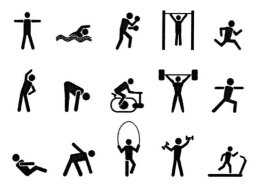

When women start exercising, their targets are to condition and obtain shape/curves and following this program will certainly reveal these.

In this program, you will decrease the reps from the initial number you complete and then increase the pounds as you move on. The number of sets will remain the same, but the number of reps changes over time.

Weeks 1-4

In this week, lifting will be at the 8-12 rep range. Meaning, you would want to complete a minimum of 8 reps, but not go over 12 reps for every set. If for instance, you are not able to finish 8 reps, the weight must be too heavy and you must lower the load. If you are able to perform more than 12 reps, the weight is too light and you must add more.

Monday- Upper Body A
- Bench Press   3 sets of 8-12 reps
- Bent Over Row   3 sets of 8-12 reps

- DB Shoulder Press   3   sets   of   8-12 reps
- Lying Tricep Extension   3   sets   of   8-12 reps
- Barbell or DB Curl   3   sets   of   8-12 reps

Tuesday Lower Body A

- Squat   3   sets   of   8-12 reps
- Stiff Leg Deadlift   3   sets   of   8-12 reps
- Leg Extension   3   sets   of   8-12 reps
- Leg Curl   3   sets   of   8-12 reps
- Standing Calf Raise   3   sets   of   8-12 reps
- Abs
- Lying Leg Raise   3   sets   of   10-15 reps
- Swiss Ball Crunch   3   sets   of   10-15 reps

Thursday- Upper Body B

- Dips   3   sets   of   8-12 reps

Bodybuilding For Women

- Pull Ups   3   sets   of   8-12 reps
- DB Side Lateral   3   sets   of   8-12 reps
- Tricep Pressdown   3   sets   of   8-12 reps
- Cable Curl   3   sets   of   8-12 reps

Friday- Lower Body B

- Deadlift   3 sets of 8-12 reps
- Leg Press   3 sets of 8-12 reps
- Lunges   3 sets of 8-12 reps
- Seated Calf Raise   3 sets of 8-12 reps
- Db Shrugs (Optional)   3 sets of 8-12 reps

Abs

- Incline Crunch   3 sets of 10-15 reps
- Back Extension   3 sets of 10-15 reps

**Rest Periods : 1 minute

Weeks 5-8

In this week, lifting will be at 6-8 rep range. Meaning, you want to finish 6 reps minimum, but not more than 8 reps for every set. If you are not able to finish 6 reps, the load is too heavy and you must decrease the weight. If you are able to perform more than 8 reps, the load is too light and you must increase the weight.

Monday- Upper Body A
- Bench Press   3 sets of 6-8 reps
- Bent Over Row   3 sets of 6-8 reps
- DB Shoulder Press   3 sets of 6-8 reps
- Lying Tricep Extension   3 sets of 6-8 reps
- Barbell ir DB Curl   3 sets of 6-8 reps

Tuesday Lower Body A
- Squat   3 sets of 6-8 reps
- Stiff Leg Deadlift   3 sets of 6-8 reps
- Leg Extension   3 sets of 6-8 reps
- Leg Curl   3 sets of 6-8 reps
- Standing Calf Raise   3 sets of 6-8 reps

Abs
- Lying Leg Raise   3 sets of 10-15 reps

- Swiss Ball Crunch   3 sets of 10-15 reps

Thursday- Upper Body B

- Dips	3 sets of 6-8 reps
- Pull Ups	3 sets of 6-8 reps
- DB Side Lateral	3 sets of 6-8 reps
- Tricep Pressdown	3 sets of 6-8 reps
- Cable Curl	3 sets of 6-8 reps

Friday- Lower Body B

- Deadlift	3 sets of 6-8 reps
- Leg Press	3 sets of 6-8 reps
- Lunges	3 sets of 6-8 reps
- Seated Calf Raise	3 sets of 6-8 reps
- Db Shrugs (Optional)	3 sets of 6-8 reps

Abs

- Incline Crunch	3 sets of 10-15 reps
- Back Extension	3 sets of 10-15 reps

**Rest Periods : 90 seconds

Weeks 9-12

In this week, lifting will be at 4-6 rep range. Meaning, you would like to finish a minimum of 4 reps but not more than 6 reps for every set. If you are unable to finish 4 reps, the weight is too heavy and must be decreased. If you are able to complete more than 6 reps, the load is too light and you must increase the weight.

Monday- Upper Body A

- Bench Press	3 sets of 4-6 reps
- Bent Over Row	3 sets of 4-6 reps
- DB Shoulder Press	3 sets of 4-6 reps
- Lying Tricep Extension	3 sets of 4-6 reps
- Barbell ir DB Curl	3 sets of 4-6 reps

Tuesday Lower Body A

- Squat	3 sets of 4-6 reps
- Stiff Leg Deadlift	3 sets of 4-6 reps
- Leg Extension	3 sets of 4-6 reps
- Leg Curl	3 sets of 4-6 reps
- Standing Calf Raise	3 sets of 4-6 reps
Abs	
- Lying Leg Raise	3 sets of 10-15 reps
- Swiss Ball Crunch	3 sets of 10-15 reps

Thursday- Upper Body B

- Dips	3 sets of 4-6 reps
- Pull Ups	3 sets of 4-6 reps
- DB Side Lateral	3 sets of 4-6 reps
- Tricep Pressdown	3 sets of 4-6 reps
- Cable Curl	3 sets of 4-6 reps

Friday- Lower Body B

- Deadlift	3 sets of 4-6 reps
- Leg Press	3 sets of 4-6 reps
- Lunges	3 sets of 4-6 reps
- Seated Calf Raise	3 sets of 4-6 reps
- Db Shrugs (Optional)	3 sets of 4-6 reps

Abs

- Incline Crunch reps	3 sets of 10-15
- Back Extension reps	3 sets of 10-15

**Rest Periods : 2 minutes

The weeks during this program will be very challenging, but eventually deliver excellent results.

Exercise Guidelines

Maintain strict form on all movements

We have stressed how essential it is to keep a proper form on all activities. This means stabilizing your body and contracting your abdominals so you are focused on one muscle group at a time. For example, when doing a standing weights curl, tighten your abs and do not rock or turn the weight. By tightening your abdominals, you maintain your body and protect against momentum. This will also work your abs while protecting your back from injury.

Do the right Warm-Up

You need to perform 1-3 sets of warm-ups prior to working on a particular muscle of the body. For example, when doing a bench press with 85 pounds, do a warm-up set with 45 pounds (or with just the bar) and afterwards a set with 65 pounds, before attempting to bench press 85 pounds.

Rest in between Sets

I suggest a period of 60-120 secs of rest in between sets. This enables your body to

Bodybuilding For Women

regain several of its ATPs, but it's not too long that you lose the rhythm of the workout. Remember, your goal is to be in the weight room for thirty to forty-five minutes.

I missed a workout, what should I do?

No worries! People are busy and tend to miss a day here and there, but there is a fix for that. All you have to do is get back on track. Do not avoid exercise! You have three off days weekly. If you miss Tuesday's exercise then attempt to do it on Wednesday and afterwards go back to your regular schedule.

ABOUT THE AUTHOR

As a writer and fitness instructor, Yvette Green reaches out to women all over the globe to help them achieve optimum health. Yvette started body building after the birth of her third child. The results of child birth on her body did not appeal to her so she worked her way through to toning her body as it was before pregnancy.

She was a success! Body building not only toned and sculpted her muscles; it improved her health and made her more resistant to illness. She started encouraging other mothers to begin body building workouts and soon the whole gym was filled with her family and friends.

A natural leader, she ventured to become a fitness instructor. Yvette went through extensive training, programs and seminars focused on health and fitness. She recently opened her own gym which is located in her backyard. Her students are her neighbors and other locals from neighboring areas.

Bodybuilding For Women

She feels good to be a healthy, physically fit mom and she wants to share her knowledge and encourage other moms to feel and become beautiful, inside and out.

CPSIA information can be obtained at www.ICGtesting.com
Printed in the USA
BVOW05s1723301114

377313BV00007B/24/P